Walter Pierpaoli

My Happy Patients
Letters to Walter Pierpaoli

INTERBION Foundation

Walter Pierpaoli

This book brings together some of the letters received by Walter Pierpaoli over recent years. The texts have undergone those adjustments and corrections that are required for the purposes of publication. The editor has sent requests to the authors for disclaimers and made all possible attempts to obtain written consent prior to publication. The letters, in any case, have been published anonymously.

The editor thanks Valerio Di Nicola for the afterword.

The drawings in this volume are by Lucio Marzano.

INTERBION Foundation for Basic Biomedical Research
CH-6595 Riazzino
Switzerland

ISBN/EAN: 978-1-326-01926-6

Foreword

Dear Friends, since life is skillfully made complicated by those who do not understand it, let us get out of that trap and leap joyfully into the rotating vortex, knowing that we are sure to come out of it safe and sound. I spent over forty years observing rats and mice – not, unfortunately, in their natural surroundings, but at least without arousing anxiety and pain in those dear little creatures that were born and grew up in confinement. Aware that I had a lot to learn from these mammals, I tried to understand how on earth they develop diseases in exactly the same way as happens in the human mammal. In this long research path, partly illustrated in the 1995 American best-seller *The Melatonin Miracle*, I conducted an endless series of experiments based, as well as on numerical evidence and statistics, mainly on my own intuition. I would say that a fundamental breakthrough – a breakthrough that led me to my current study of medicine – happened when I conducted an extraordinarily simple experiment, but one that nobody had ever thought of or carried out before. This study was subsequently published with the title *Pharmacological control of the hormonally mediated immune response* (in the volume *Psychoneuroimmunology*, edited by R. Ader, Academic Press, New York 1981, pp. 405-428). I already realised back then the role of the day-night rhythm on hormone variations and consequently, on the natural immunity controlled by them. I put 10 young female mice under the light of a lamp, day and night, in the company of a male. I kept the cages in the same laboratory to facilitate control and observation of them. Still under the light, the females gave birth and suckled their young. When these became adult without showing any alteration, the second generation was likewise kept under permanent light. I then continued the same treatment without noting anything until the third generation. Fortunately I went on with the experiment, and confirmed my conviction that changing the circadian rhythm – with a real alteration in the genes controlling it in the brain, or even the eradication of them – would take a very long time. And then I was to have another, more important confirmation: that the circadian rhythm, precisely because of the very long times needed to upset it, must be really *fundamental* for life.

My patience was rewarded by an extraordinary observation. In the fourth generation, I saw that the new-born mice did not grow normally: they were altered, dystrophic and appeared prematurely aged. I was able to verify that their thymus, the gland on which immunity is based, was atrophic and the immune response of the antibodies was insufficient. In short, the abolition of circadian rhythms, occurring in mice kept under permanent light after four generations, had caused *premature ageing*. This simple experiment supported my intuition, derived from two decades of experiments in endocrinology and immunology: day-night circadian rhythms control the synthesis and the release of *growth-type and thyroid-type hormones*, essential for somatic development and for the health of the immune system.

The simple experiment was, in fact, revolutionary, offering once again a confirmation, at the highest level, of the fact that the truth is right before our eyes every day, but we do not see it.

As we may easily understand, these observations back in the late 1970s already showed clearly how maintaining hormonal circadian rhythms constitutes a *sine qua non* for disease prevention. Many more years – and many more discoveries – have gone by, and now I can talk, more appropriately, of *maintaining hormonal inter-synchronization* to describe the constant and precise interaction of hormones over 24 hours: *the basis of health.*

In this way and very gradually, I approached the mysterious (and sometimes even considered as useless) pineal gland, which at night produces a strange indolamine whose synthesis requires two important enzyme passages, acetylation and methylation. In 2014, it seems almost impossible that we do not understand how the rhythm of the pineal gland is the signal for growth, fertility and ageing processes in humans. However, before conducting the night-time administration of melatonin to 18-month-old mice, many other experiments were needed, all of which were illustrated in dozens of publications. Indeed, the logic appears to be foreign and inaccessible to many people who get bogged down in the details and expatiate at length, in never-ending disquisitions of a specialist nature on genetics, molecular biology, endocrinology and immunology. In actual fact, there is only the planetary cosmic logic that has generated life: *rotational cycles.*

I am explaining this in order to illustrate how the maintenance and restructuring of central rhythms leads inevitably to the prevention of diseases and to a *programmed* organic decay, called ageing. This gently brings us to the end of our lifecycle and to the final pineal message: you die at between 110 and 130 years. This is the real life-program of the human mammal.

Walter Pierpaoli

Around 20 years ago I wrote the following comment: *To age or not to age: this is Hamlet's dilemma. What is ageing?* I am sure that there is only one type of ageing and not several. I mean that the biological process of ageing is similar and repetitive for all homeothermic (warm-blooded) mammals. It is an evolutionary program in the brain that follows very precise, inescapable rules. These rules are hereditary and unrelenting. However, they are not a mysterious dogma and can be interpreted and modified. Unfortunately for us, many people in the past thought and still think that the inversion of ageing is a ridiculous, blasphemous idea. Now we say: growth can be slowed down and modified, fertility can be anticipated or delayed. It is the pituitary hormones that control growth and fertility. Therefore, why should we not be able to modify the ageing program?

I think the explanations for this are of various kinds, except for being logical and scientific. Logical thought and scientific evidence contrast violently with the narrow-mindedness of those who, with their various interests, oppose the idea that ageing can be retarded and could even be reversible. This reality would deprive many of their 'little gardens' where they grow ideas of 'low-calorie diets', 'anti-oxidants', 'telomeres', 'enzymes', 'essential ions' and other marvellous new molecules and lots more besides. However, there is an extraordinary simplicity inherent in Nature, even though it seems foreign to the human brain. Thus many presumed anti-ageing prophets or pioneers have unfortunately died before they can demonstrate they are right! I have known some of them; now we take up the challenge.

Why, if diseases are not prevented, is it in any way possible to cure them?

It is absurdly simple! In the three main groups of diseases that relentlessly attack the world and that afflicted *My happy patients*, we can number the following: cardiovascular diseases caused by rapid or progressive sclerosis of the arteries, be they capillary, arteriolar or large vessel (for example the aorta), in any area of the body (these are around 60% of the total deaths); cancers (another good 30% of the total deaths); and then neurodegenerative diseases such as Parkinson's, multiple sclerosis, motor neurone and autoimmune diseases, almost always triggered with a primary viral or bacterial infective component.

We must reflect. In all the pathologies we considered which afflicted *My happy patients,* there is a common denominator that makes the therapy even more logical. This, as I have tried to describe in a few lines above, is a *central hormonal de-synchronization with consequent alteration in the oxidative metabolism, a collapse of viral and delayed immune control and the beginning of a vicious cycle, with a multitude of symptoms that hide, to the point of 'forgetting', the neuroendocrine-immune origin of the pathology.*

My therapeutic interventions – developed progressively since 1996 when I resumed treating patients again – have taken advantage of the possibility of restoring biological hormonal circadian rhythms starting from the pituitary gland and from the dreadful thyroid deficiency that affects almost all the population. I soon noticed that the pathologies, with widely varying names and definitions, have, in fact, one common root: a genetically inherited or acquired alteration leading inevitably to a progression of cancerous or degenerative pathologies (atherosclerosis). Striking examples are the powerful cancerogenous action of the prolactin pituitary hormones, TSH and to a lesser extent, the growth (somatotropic) hormone. But the main element, by a long way, is a state of hypothyroidism that demolishes the immune resistance system and generates all sorts of pathologies. There is a hitherto

7

unknown state that was discovered, studied and carefully examined by me, which is at the basis of the development of all cardiovascular diseases and which I have defined as *pituitary hypothyroidism*, easily identifiable by the imbalance in temperature control and by low TSH, FT3 and FT4 values. Unfortunately the values given by laboratory tests are totally unreliable. The state of relative thyroid inactivity consequent on TSH pituitary deficiency is the prime cause of the process of arteriosclerosis.

To summarise: each type of pathology involves an alteration in hormonal rhythms. In the vast majority of cases they go back to the pituitary gland and to the thyroid, which is always susceptible to recovery *upstream* with the appropriate administration of T3 and T4 thyroid hormones. When the hormonal circadian rhythms are re-established they gradually ensure a total recovery of body equilibrium. We have even forgotten that the pituitary hormones are voluminous proteins and that therefore, the thyroid hormone T3 has an essential role in synthesising them.

I would like to conclude with a more obvious account of the miracles of hormones during seasonal cycles, by referring to that great masterpiece of classical Roman literature by an unknown author. It takes us back to the Catania Plain, underneath Mount Etna, into an ancient, ideal world, in harmony with Nature and Procreation: the poem *Pervigilium Veneris*.

Cras amet qui numquam amavit quique amavit cras amet!
Ver novum, ver iam canorum; vere natus orbis est,
Vere concordant amores, vere nubunt alites,

Et nemus comam resolvit de maritis imbribus.
Cras amorum copulatrix inter umbras arborum
Implicat casas virentis de flagello myrteo,
Cras Dione iura dicit fulta sublimi throno.
Cras amet qui numquam amavit…

(Love tomorrow, loveless ones! And you who have loved,
love tomorrow!
Spring is now here, spring full of songs; the world was born
in spring,
Lovers are happy together, the birds mate in spring
And the plants let their hair down after marital showers.
Tomorrow the great Matchmaker will build green shelters
with myrtle leaves under the shade of the trees:
Tomorrow Venus is in charge, upon her heavenly throne.
Love tomorrow, loveless ones! And you who have loved,
love tomorrow!)

What more fitting message could there be to help us understand the essence of *My happy patients*?

Walter Pierpaoli

Happy Patients
Letters to Walter Pierpaoli

Walter Pierpaoli

I.   The key of life

Dear Doctor Pierpaoli,

I am writing to you like this because I have seen some of your interviews on YouTube and you seemed to me to be an extremely humble person full of ideas … a wonderful person, a scientist who considers research to be a mission aimed at people's wellbeing and not just for making money. I respect people who have the courage to swim against the tide. Now I'll explain the reasons for this message. I am a 40-year-old woman. I live in B. and since I was a small child (since I was 8-10 years of age) I have been suffering from psychological problems which, with the passing of time, have become more and more oppressive. I have been treated by psychologists, psychiatrists and all the other possible professionals. They suggested I had (if I have to use their diagnostic vocabulary) bipolar disorder, obsessive-compulsive syndrome, bulimia with vomiting, social phobia, and agoraphobia. I won't go on. I would define it as a deep sadness in my soul, a prison without bars that made my life hell. In all these years my body lived, continuously, only at very high levels of anxiety and restlessness so that any attempt to create anything or simply to live a normal life became impossible for me. My mind was obsessive... but capable of enormous vitality and of intense, positive energy, able to be amazed and to marvel at the magnificence of our world. I consider myself as an infinite spirit destined to die in an unnatural finiteness... a mind avid for knowledge that is unable to satisfy this voracious hunger because it is too unstable...

To come to the point: I started to take your melatonin around two weeks ago. I was very impressed by your research: through a strange coincidence, I was looking into the pineal gland as an organ with very deep spiritual implications. I considered your discoveries extremely well-founded and illuminating. The anxiety that had dogged me for more than twenty years seems to have completely disappeared. It was so ingrained in my perceptions that it was like losing a part of myself. I wondered if it was the power of suggestion. I will go on taking it mainly because I have had such good results in such a short time and this has given me a real enthusiasm for it. I intend to make as many people as possible (who, like me, suffer from this invisible disease) aware of the results they could achieve without ruining their lives with drugs.

Thank you for giving me a serenity that was denied to me for too many years.

A.

Walter Pierpaoli

II.   Skin-rash defeated

Dear Doctor,

It is with great joy that I write to you to let you know that one of my problems (cold urticaria, which was restricting my life considerably: after just fifteen minutes of exposure to the cold, I had to rush to find shelter by going into a warm environment to make the redness of my skin, which was similar to a scald, fade away), has been solved. Now I go out confidently (within limits, of course!) without any trouble, and I can assure you that it seems like a dream because I had suffered from this for fifteen years.

I would say that, all in all, I feel fine, although I have been suffering slightly, for about two weeks now, from feelings of instability (especially in the mornings). Luckily, these are not attacks of dizziness as happened in the past, but they cause a sense of disorientation, restlessness and difficulty in concentration: if I take my blood pressure I find that compared with the evenings (60-70/110-120) the values are higher (from 75-80/130-140) with a pulse of up to 95... What is causing this, in your opinion? Could it be the cold or the menopause? Why do I still frequently have hot flushes with sweating? I hope very much to come through this, as happened with the skin rash.

I have been following your treatment for almost eight months now, and I will be finishing the fourth kit in a few days. Have I reached the maintenance phase? I look forward to receiving your instructions.

Thank you so much for what you are doing.

A. F.

Walter Pierpaoli

III.   The end of an ordeal

I apologise for the delay in writing these lines, which re-surface from my sad recollections. It was right back in November 1996 when I, a bold youngster, found I had uveitis in my right eye. It was a real ordeal to find a diagnosis for it and then, the following summer, after several hospital stays and lots of dead-ends, on the advice of some oculists I went to a clinic in Switzerland where, after a simple examination, they sent me home with a request for a bronchoscopy, to establish whether it was sarcoidosis or Behçet's disease.

The answer was the latter and my ordeal (not only mine, but also my family's) started from there. I had some interbulbar infiltrations in the right eye, in Padua, with the sole result that the recidivating uveitis was seen to disappear – but so did my sight in that eye, *completely*.

In the following years I resumed normal life. I got married and in January 1999 the new ordeal started. At home, when I woke up from my afternoon nap, my wife told me my right eye was completely distorted. Several hospital stays followed, with scanty results, cortisone treatment over and over again and my physical condition ruined. I was lucky enough to become a father, but a few months later, in September 1999, I had two collapsed vertebrae.

It was in January 2001 that I heard about you and your work, thanks to mutual friends and my uncle, who was also devastated by this illness and who took an interest in my plight.

I started your treatment and we began to get to know each other. During one of my frequent hospital stays in the subsequent months, the spinal column X-rays showed (quite miraculously!) that the fractures to the vertebrae had reset themselves. Today, the situation is completely different and if I did not have stretch marks on my arms and abdomen I would not even remember that twelve years ago I was more dead than alive. I will always be grateful to you for all you did.

A. B.

IV.   No more panic attacks!

Dear Doctor Pierpaoli,

I wanted to bring you up to date on the progress of my therapy: in the last two months, in spite of some particular personal difficulties, your therapy has helped me to feel more alive again and the panic attacks are decreasing in number and intensity. Having used the various products freely for less than one month, I would like to ask you how I should proceed and if I should continue with the same kit that is bringing me benefits: can you give the prescription to the pharmacy?

I would also like to know if we will meet again in September and if I should have tests done again before that appointment.

With gratitude and great respect, I remain,

Yours sincerely,

A.C.

ACCIDENT AND EMERGENCY

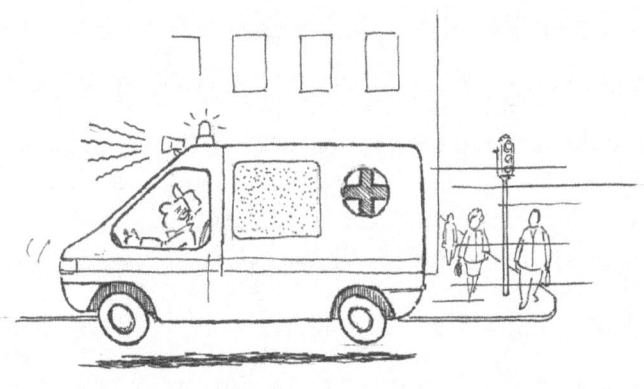

1.

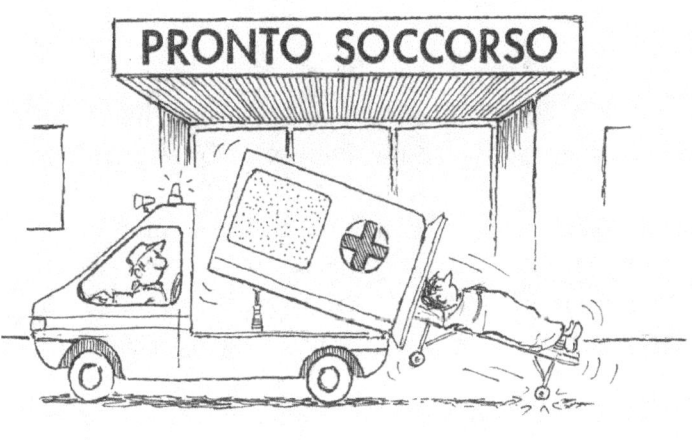

2.

Walter Pierpaoli

V.   Treating premature menopause

Dear Doctor Pierpaoli,

I would like to inform you that after an approximately five-year absence of menstruation, I had my period again last Friday. I am using the progesterone cream every evening. Everything else is going well.
Thank you again for your help!
Regards.

A.G.

*

I am writing to bring you up to date on my state of health. I am enclosing the analyses, (the white blood cells have decreased considerably) and the abdominal ultrasound, (the inflammation has returned). My abdominal swelling has gone down and the only problem is having to go frequently to the toilet. I have finished the whole box of acidophilus tablets: should I continue to take them?
I look forward with confidence, as always, to hearing from you.
Yours sincerely,

A.G.

***

What more can you ask? I would still continue with the acidophilus tablets. These pathologies are cured if one does not end up in the hands of 'experts', 'dietologists' and other 'nothingologists' and start again eating everything and educating your stomach and intestine – even allowing it to get shaken up and to rumble! We are made up of pipes anyway, aren't we?

With best wishes,

Walter Pierpaoli

Walter Pierpaoli

VI.   Cancer defeated

Dear Doctor,

I expect you have already left. It is a pity that my life has taken a wrong turning... I confess that I am a failed dentist. I have fallen back on being a hygienist, although I was in fact enrolled in dentistry; fate, however, played a mean trick on me...

I took my mother for a check-up with an oncologist. The tumour markers had gone down from 186 to 117! The oncologist told me with a smile 'You see...the treatment works!'

What could I say? Hooray!

Would you be so kind, when you have time, to prescribe the new medicines for me. We are coming to see you in October and I will bring the new tests and my clinical record (as you will remember, I have Addison's disease).

With best wishes,
Yours sincerely,

A.N.

VII. A new life

Dear Doctor Pierpaoli,

Both my husband and I have finished the therapy! My name is *D.A.*, and I am taking the second kit and I feel really well, as though I were 10 years younger: my headaches and aching bones have gone away! I will leave it to you to tell me what I should do... My husband, *A*. has various cardio-circulatory problems: we recently gave up the cardio-aspirin. We thank you so much, and wish you good health and a long life: everything has been of benefit to us, too! Thank you again.

D.A.

Walter Pierpaoli

ORTHOPAEDICS

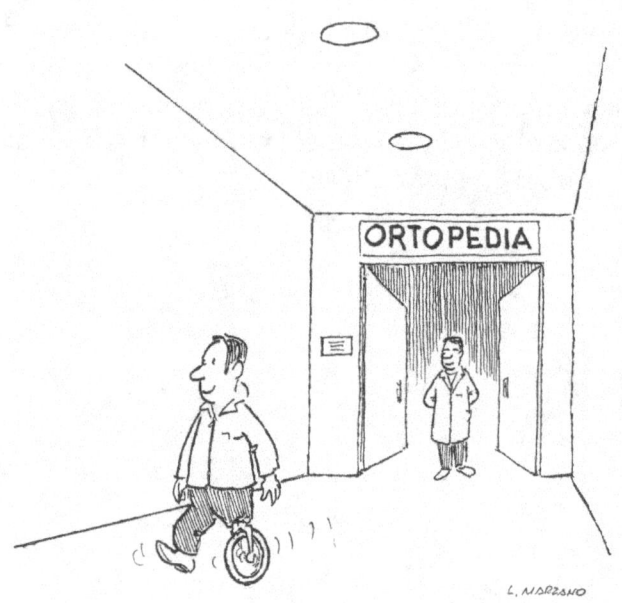

VIII. Energy and vitality thanks to melatonin

Dear Dr. Pierpaoli,

My name is *B*, and I am the daughter of Mr. *M*. I hope you are well.

I must thank you so much; your treatment is doing me a lot of good. I have a new-found energy and thanks to the melatonin I am actually able to sleep much better. I will finish the first two months' treatment on 6 November and then I would like to know from you what I should do: would it be useful for me to have new blood tests? Should I continue the treatment using the same kit and the same doses? Or should I make some alterations? Please would you tell me as soon as possible how I should proceed, so that I can let Dr. *C.* know and have everything prepared for me before I finish the kit I am using.

Thank you in advance for your help. I wish you a pleasant evening! Best wishes also from my husband and my little Nicolò.

I look forward to hearing from you,

B.M.

IX.   I feel well!

Dear Dr. Pierpaoli,

My name is *B.*; we met in the Pesaro consulting rooms and I started your treatment. Apart from the first few days when I had some headache and acidity problems, I then got on fine with it and felt much better. Now my vitality is considerably improved and I feel well! Since the kit you prescribed me is for two months, I wanted to know what I should do, whether I should take the same medicines or if I should have tests. Thank you in advance; I look forward to hearing from you.
      Yours sincerely,

B.B.

X. New-found vitality, and fertility

Dear Doctor Pierpaoli,

I am writing to let you know that I have almost finished the first two months of the treatment you prescribed for me following our meeting here in P., and I therefore need a new prescription.

I can tell you that I generally feel much better; my temperature is constantly between 36.1 and 36.2, I am finally sleeping very well and I wake up with an energy I had never had before; I also realise that I can cope better with the harsh temperatures at this time of year, compared with previous years, and that I have a good complexion. And I have not yet felt any of the seasonal ailments (influenza, cold, cough, etc.) that I have always suffered from.

The only thing I cannot understand is why, ever since I have been taking the capsules, my intestine has not been working more regularly as it did before. In fact, a short time (15-20 minutes) after swallowing the capsules I often have stomach-ache. How can I correct this problem? Regarding the annoying itching on the scrotum which I talked to you about, I can confirm that, although it has not disappeared, it has anyway improved considerably and I have also noted that it varies according to my state of mind. For example, if it happens to be a day or a situation that causes stress, anxiety or in any case an uneasy state of mind, the irritation is more acute, while on days when I feel calm, the itching disappears almost entirely. Is this a coincidence or could the two things be associated?

Walter Pierpaoli

One last thing, but one which I think will require more time, concerns the 'baby-question'.
In spite of our attempts during this last month, we have still not been successful. I would ask you therefore to kindly let me know how to proceed, and if I should have the tests done again.

I look forward to hearing from you.
With best wishes,

C.V.

***

Dear *C.,*

Thank you for bringing me up to date. I am thinking about your case and I will arrange with Doctor *C.* I am sure we will arrive at the perfect balance, which also requires good sense and collaboration on the part of the patient. I think that you are taking the capsules *during meals* and not on an empty stomach, which would explain the problems. My treatment, on the other hand, is useful to reactivate gastro-intestinal muscles.

Regarding the baby, we do not have to wait until Divine Providence sees to it, as it has plenty of other things to do...

With kind regards and best wishes to you and your family,

Walter Pierpaoli

***

Dear Doctor,

Thank you for your quick reply. I do, in fact, take the capsules just before breakfast (10/15 minutes), at lunchtime while I am eating (during lunch) and in the evening during dinner, except for the melatonin, which I take about 30 minutes before going to bed. I probably wrongly interpreted the information about when to take them, as given on the instruction sheet, and I will immediately go and look at it again to correct this problem. I am completely optimistic about achieving the perfect balance and there is full collaboration on my part and also respect for you, so I will scrupulously follow all the advice I receive from you.

For this very reason, since I cannot trust in Divine Providence, what can I do?

With very best wishes to you and your family, too.

C.V.

* * *

Trust me: I have a special link. Enhance your diet with fats. They are highly important for fertility. With very best wishes,

Walter Pierpaoli

Walter Pierpaoli

* * *

Dear Doctor,

I am writing to let you know that I have almost finished the second six-month period of treatment and everything is going really well. I continue to feel all the benefits I was talking about in my previous email and all the problems I had before are starting to become a bad dream as the days go by.
I would therefore ask you kindly to let me know how I should proceed.
Have a good day.
With best wishes,

C.V.

* * *

Dear C.,

I was very glad to hear your news. I am away at the moment and will look into things as soon as I return.
With best wishes,

Walter Pierpaoli

* * *

Dear Doctor,

I am writing to thank you and let you know about the immense happiness that has filled our lives since we discovered that *C.* will give birth soon (on around 12 November) to our long-awaited baby.

There are no words to describe our gratitude and we can simply thank you from the bottom of our hearts.

I would like to take this opportunity also to tell you that in around 8 days' time I will have finished the six-month treatment and I would ask you kindly to arrange things with Doctor *C.*

With our great respect and affection,

C.& C.

I am so happy for you! And it is also my reward, don't you think? I will arrange things.

With best wishes,

Walter Pierpaoli

* * *

Absolutely!!!
Thank you and have a good day,

C.V.

Walter Pierpaoli

XI. Treating hepatitis

Dear Doctor Pierpaoli,

I would like to thank you from the bottom of my heart for having recommended your melatonin formula to me for treating my chronic hepatitis. I want to tell you that, after a few months of therapy with your zinc + selenium + melatonin, the enzyme values have completely returned to normal. The most significant data, however, lies in the fact that I feel much better and less tired, after so many years spent in the dark and discouraged. Even the state of my mood is improving day by day. At the hepatology centre, where I go every six months for a check-up, they have been amazed at the values for my blood, asking me what I do apart from not drinking alcohol: I have preferred to keep quiet, as they have been terrorising me for years because I have always refused their treatment with interferon and ribavirin. And so, to make absolutely sure, they subjected me to a non-invasive, Fibroscan examination, to see the fibrotic state of my liver. Well, this examination gave a result of 7.4, which indicates a normal level of elasticity in my liver tissue. As things stood, they told me to come back in a year, but I am sure that I will get better and better, and this is thanks to you, because you gave me the hope to believe in life as the greatest value. I apologise if I have gone on about it a bit too long, but I was keen to relate this wonderful happening to you!

Ci.C.

Dear Doctor Pierpaoli,

I am writing to you once again, with great enthusiasm, to thank you from the bottom of my heart, since, by taking your zinc + selenium + melatonin formula, my life has improved significantly, both from a general point of view and in terms of my liver. Well, I did the blood tests again for the periodic liver check and the general picture is very satisfactory. A year ago, the specialist who is looking after my case wanted to have me follow the traditional treatment with interferon and ribavirin. I refused because of the serious side-effects, even though he told me that I could be finally cured. Seeing that the values for hepatic enzymes had gone down he was rather perplexed, as I am not following any specific treatment for my pathology. I told him that I had been taking melatonin for three months, and had noticed less tiredness and more calm. – while they have always terrified me with the idea that I will certainly suffer from cirrhosis, even though the ultrasounds only show a moderate echo-structural dishomogeneity due to the disease, with biliar, pancreatic and splenetic function normal. I can never understand why the doctors do not really ascertain the curative power of melatonin in the formula devised and experimented by you over so many years of research. Is it possible that they are not honest and objective when they pronounce themselves in favour of the possibility of a therapy for those who suffer? Personally, I believe that I have a chance to recover. Thank you, Doctor; mine is just one humble testimony. I have hopes that my disease can be combated effectively with the use of your melatonin. May God bless you always! And I apologise for making you waste your valuable time every now and then.

Ci.C.

Dear Doctor Pierpaoli,

I am sorry for writing to you occasionally; however, I have great faith in you because, as well as being a great luminary in the study of melatonin, you are a good-hearted person. I have been taking your product, in fact, for a long time for my chronic hepatitis C, with positive results for my health in general, (I have never felt so well, whereas before I was always very tired). Now I feel calmer because, thanks to you, I have understood how important this substance is for a healthy balance, and I also recommend my friends to take your melatonin, instead of the many others on sale that they were aware of. I tell them about my positive experience since I have been taking your melatonin with zinc and selenium. Now, Doctor, I would like to ask you if I can take two tablets instead of one, since one evening, when I took two of them by mistake, I felt its benefits more strongly in the morning and during the day. Finally, one more important question which I would like to bring to your attention and try your patience with: is it true that taking melatonin has led to a reduction in the fibrotic process of the liver in guinea-pigs, also showing an improvement in the response of hepatic parameters? Thank you very much for your kindness; I look forward to hearing from you.

May God bless you always, for the great gift you have given to humankind!

Ci.C.

XII. I have started to live again

Dear Doctor,

I am writing because I am coming to the end of your last prescription for kit no. 3. Thank you again for all the good that I have had from your treatment; I do not remember feeling so healthy for years, or even decades.

I am only sorry not to be able to thank you in person, although I hope to meet you if you should visit here in T.

I would ask you kindly for instructions to continue with the treatment, and am at your disposal for any information you should consider necessary.

Thank you for having taken care of me. Thank you also on behalf of my family, who can now, because of my improved state of health, count on having in me a contented family-member.

I wish you all the best,
Kind regards,

Ci.C.

XIII. Just a matter of luck?

Dear Doctor Pierpaoli,

Here are the results of the tests: the doctor did not believe her eyes, she wanted me to repeat them and they are exceptional. You see, Doctor, the most difficult thing when one decides to come to you for treatment and one is cured, is fighting with one's family doctor. This is why I have decided not to go to her any more, with the additional reason that I have not needed to, since you have had me in your care. Today, however, doctors are computerized and do not miss a thing.

	21/02/09	26/08/09
Glycaemia	237	145
Triglycerides	195	135
Total cholesterol	299	198
Ldl cholesterol	180	140
Hdl cholesterol	52	31
Glycos. Haemoglobin	9.2	7.6

It is a great result and I am delighted. I will never be able to thank you enough. I can imagine how much patience you have to have with us. I wish you all the best from life.

D.B.

Walter Pierpaoli

XIV. New energy!

Dear Doctor,

Did you have a good Christmas? I am sure you did! I am writing to you for some advice. As you will remember, I started your treatment at the end of April 2008 with a 'kit 2', and then went on with two 'kit 4s'. Since October, following your advice, I continued only with a whole Thyroid IBSA 125 in the morning and a melatonin in the evening.

The treatment has brought results: I have lost a few excess kilos, my skin has improved, and so has my diet and my energy in the mornings – and for this I thank you very much indeed; it is all thanks to you!

However, for about a month now, I have been waking up with some fairly distinct, itchy red marks on various parts of my body (arms, legs, ankles, sides): sometimes they disappear, and sometimes they persist. It is not eczema (which I had as a child) since, when they disappear; they do not leave any trace. I would like to ask you when I should repeat the treatment (a couple of times a year, if I am not mistaken) and could you recommend some particular remedy for the problem of the marks?

I was thinking of having the complete blood tests done again around April, but I would be grateful for your confirmation on this point also.

Dear Doctor, I take this opportunity to send you my very best wishes for a new year full of great projects and peace.

With kind regards,

Cr.C.

XV. Treating an irregular menstrual cycle and period pain

Dear Doctor Pierpaoli,

I am so happy! I had my period from 10 to 15 December, and it was completely painless. It is fantastic; this had not happened to me for years... and I did not have to treat myself with absurd, disgusting remedies!

I still have a whole jar of progesterone cream, (which will therefore last me until the beginning of February, or rather, for 2 more treatment cycles of 14 days each) and tablets until 29 December, but I imagine we will 'be in touch' after that because, like me, you will want to enjoy the Christmas holidays.

Santa Claus, on my behalf (even though he arrives on Saint Lucy's day here, and my party was lovely, also because we spent it with my little one-year-old boy), will make me a present of your two books. So I will not ask you any more questions which you have already answered in full!

My heartfelt good wishes for a Happy Christmas,

E.T.

XVI. A born-again woman!

Dear Doctor Pierpaoli,

I am here to ask you again, at the end of two more months of treatment (I do not know what number kit was the last one you prescribed) how we should carry on for the next phase.

The situation is really splendid; I am a born-again woman. Just to quote the figures, I should mention that in the whole month of February I had 2 migraine attacks.

In particular, even if it is perhaps only auto-suggestion, I must tell you that I have the impression that the progesterone cream has a beneficial effect on me. For example, I had a more abundant, flowing period (while for a long time I had had minimal periods). In addition, I have found that if I apply a little of it maybe to my face when I feel the first tinglings of an attack, I can avoid it.

Apart from this, everything is fine. As you predicted, my sleep has become regular over time. I do not sleep for very many hours, but they are very restful.

I hope you are still in good form as when I saw you last. I wish you all the best for the Easter holiday, and look forward to hearing from you.

E.S.

*

Walter Pierpaoli

The only fact I should mention – and it may even be a coincidence – is that, unfortunately, since I started, I have been having annoying haemorrhoids and pimples in general, and sometimes mouth ulcers: it seems like I am, as they used to say, a bit 'overheated'. You will be able to judge better than I if there is a correlation between what you have prescribed for me and these complaints.

From what I have read in your books, I gather that administering melatonin does not always produce beneficial effects immediately in regulating sleep; in fact, to tell the truth, I might observe that my sleep is rather restless at the present time. Perhaps I am being in too much of a hurry?

I must say, however, that I am delighted to be feeling better from the migraine point of view, so that the fact of having irregular sleeping patterns is really the least of my worries.

I hope I have expressed to you, and I stress this to show how important it is, *the joy that I have in my heart and the euphoric sensation that pervades my being with this improvement, and also my deep sense of gratitude.*

E.S.

XVII. I am expecting a baby!

Dear Doctor Pierpaoli,

I have pleasure in announcing that I am expecting a baby! As always, your treatment has been effective; thank you so much.

Now the question is: what should I do? Do I have to continue with the cream? Should I change the treatment?

On Saturday I had the tests done and I think they will be ready in a week's time; as soon as I pick them up I will send them to you, but in the meantime I would like to know how I should proceed.

Thank you again.

Yours affectionately,

F.S.

Walter Pierpaoli

CHEMIST INSTANT LAXATIVES 3 MIN.

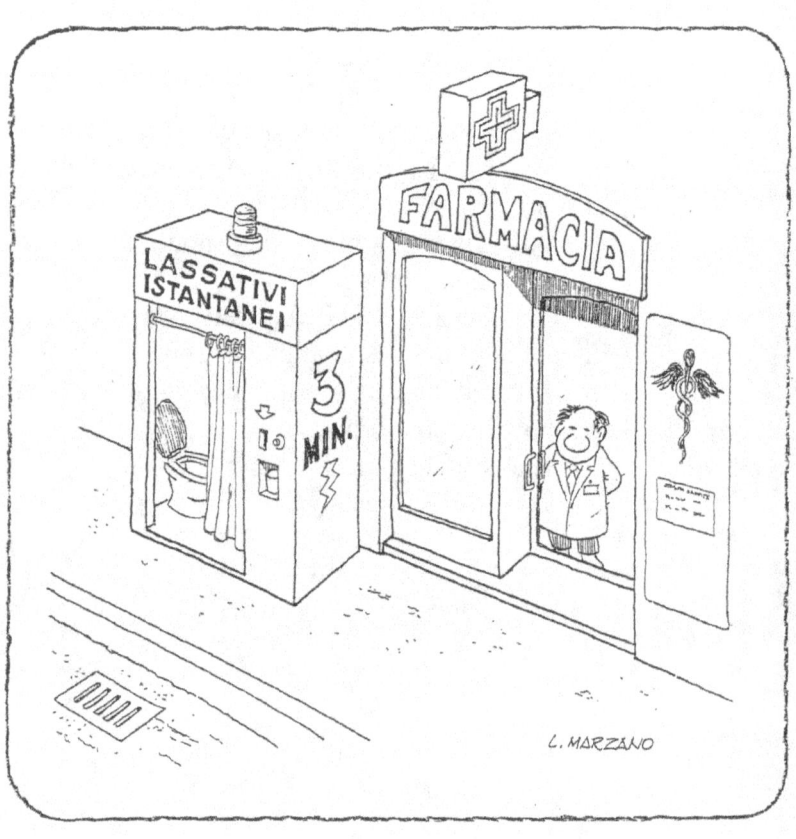

XVIII. Everybody wants to meet you!

Dear Doctor,

How are you? I hope everything is going well. I apologise for bothering you but I am writing because, having spoken about you to a lot of people, they would all like to meet you for an examination! *M.B.* and I are following your treatments regularly and day by day we feel better and better. It is as if we were reborn!

I called Ms. *I.* to make appointments with you for these people; there are four of them for now, two women and two men resident in R. There could be more later on!

I look forward to hearing news from you.

Yours sincerely,

G.C. and M.B.

Walter Pierpaoli

XIX. Miracle?

Dear Doctor,

It is with immense pleasure that I inform you that the tests for *M.G.* and *G.* are, according to the doctors, exceptional: they were absolutely amazed at the improvement achieved, which was completely unexpected.

M.G.: CD4 from 224 to 275; viral load has gone from 409 to zero;
G.: CD4 has gone from 200 to 196; viral load has gone from zero to 32.9.

Thank you very much for your help.
With best wishes,

G.F.

XX. Health regained

Dear Doctor Pierpaoli,

My name is *G.M.*, and I am a friend of *P.C.* As you already know, I started the second kit on 22 January. I wanted to let you know that for a few days now I have been feeling perfectly well, as I have never felt in my whole life before; I am satisfied, and for this I have only you to thank.

I find it incredible; this wellbeing is enabling me to find a new life, with emotions that I have never felt before and that I did not believe existed. Thank you, Doctor, you are a really amazing person.

Now, however, I am wondering if this wonderful state will last or is it only transitory?

I am a little worried about my wife, a person who has supported me up to now with a great will to help me and get me well, and who has shown great strength... She is collapsing, and I am afraid she is becoming depressed. How can we help her? Please could you give me some advice, especially as I do not want her to go through the hell I have gone through.

Please help me to help her.

With kind regards,

G.M.

Walter Pierpaoli

XXI. Happy patients

Dear Doctor,

Everything is fine here in Brescia, apart from the terrible cold. My friend *P.* is continuing the treatment and I am pleased to note that he is very active and always in a good mood; perhaps he is now convinced that he has to use a wheelchair. He always talks about your treatment to everybody who comes to see him, just in order to spite his family doctor.
Best wishes,

G.D.

* * *

Thank you for the news. We are only at the beginning and this 'Ptolemaic medicine' must come to an end. If I ever have a base in the Brescia area, we will carry out operations that cannot be imagined. Otherwise another 100 years of pharmacological holocaust will go by. Thank you for your trust.
Best wishes,

Walter Pierpaoli

* * *

Dear Doctor,

We are at the end of the treatment: everything you prescribed for us has been taken. How should we go on? I hope you will manage to contact our friend *P*.

Yours sincerely,

G.D.

Walter Pierpaoli

UROLOGY

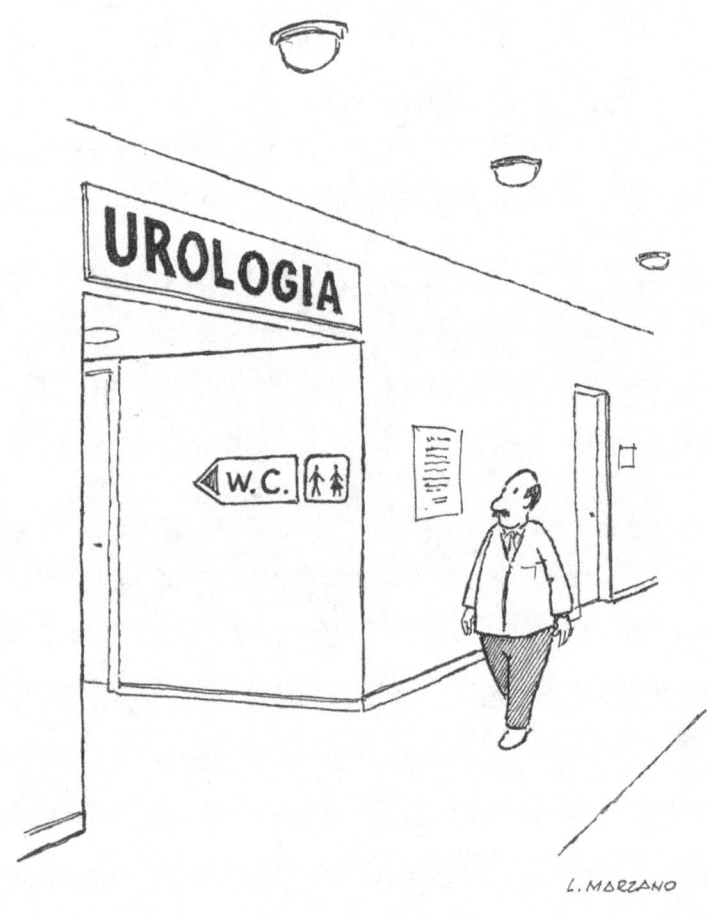

XXII. I feel younger than I did 7 years ago!

Hi Dr. Pierpaoli,

Just wanted to say that I have been taking the Melatonin ZN SE since October and have been feeling great results. For the first time in I don't know how many years, I looked forward to my birthday and didn't dread it (I turned 52 in February) and feel younger than I did 7 years ago. Also had the second period in the last 3 months, (in the fall you mentioned to me to wait at least 6 months to really see results when I mentioned I got a period right away). I also notice younger weight distribution on my body and less jowly fat along my jawline (I am a slim person, but the weight was beginning to distribute in a more middle aged way. Now it is distributing differently, all this and many other benefits.

My question: In some articles you had mentioned taking the melatonin for some periods and then going off it for a little while. Is there some type of on/off formula I can understand and follow here?

Thanks and best,

H.P.

XXIII.   Old drugs and new medicine

Dear Doctor Pierpaoli,

I am writing to let you know that I am very pleased with your treatment, which I started a month ago. I stopped taking the drugs that I had been prescribed and began with your kit and I have had no negative symptoms. I actually feel much less tired and my intestine is working very well. My menstrual cycle has been regular, and only on the second day did I have a slight sense of lethargy. It all went away very quickly. My sleep is regular and deep. I have, it is true, noted the appearance of pimples on my chin, nose and neck, which I have never had before, but what makes me happy is that after just one month's treatment my white blood-cells, after a year of continually falling, have risen a little, the haematocrit is perfectly normal and the analyses of average cell haemoglobin concentration are also satisfactory.

I have great faith in you, and this is why I would like to continue having your treatment.

I would like to know what I should do after the initial treatment prescribed by you.

Thank you very much indeed.

L.C.

VICTORIA GARAGE

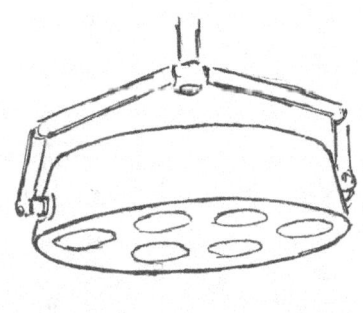

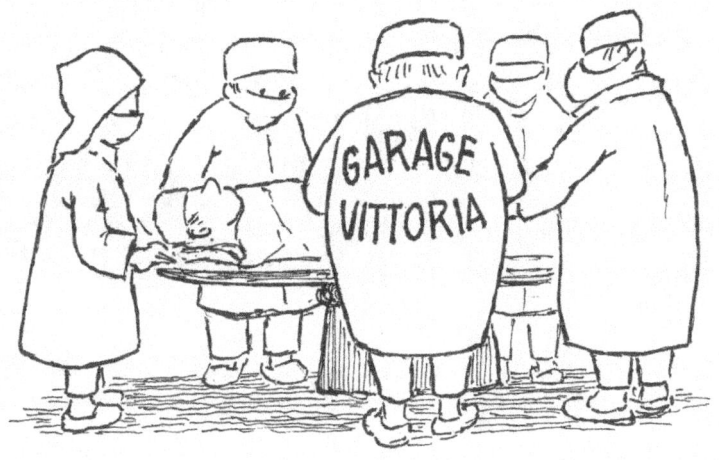

Walter Pierpaoli

XXIV. Treating premature menopause

Dear Doctor,

I have finished the third kit you prescribed for me. I have taken kit no. 4 for two months and kit no. 3 for two months and I feel fine. I would also like to inform you that this month, after being in premature menopause for more than a year, I had a regular cycle again. I would therefore like to ask you for a new prescription to continue the treatment. You could send it by fax, as last time, to the P. chemist's.

Thank you very much indeed,

L.N.

XXV. An unhoped-for help to treat epilepsy

Dear Doctor,

I saw you on TV and I tried to phone to report on my improvement and to give hope to those who are going through the same ordeal as me.

I have seen one of your videos on the Internet: you maintained that it is very important to know about one's parents' illnesses. Well, my father has glaucoma; the diagnosis goes back to 14 years ago now and he is 80 years old. It was discovered because my brother, at 40 years old and after an eye check-up, was diagnosed with glaucoma.

My mother had a cerebral ischemia and a small infarction following one of my father's epileptic attacks: he had taken an antibiotic he was allergic to.

My temperature in recent days has been as follows: 36.4; 36.3; 36.1; 36.2; 36.1; 36.2; 36.3; 36.1.

Since 5 February I have had only two attacks: I am pleased with my improvement. The neurologists tried everything, without results. And I was always told that I was a separate case.

This is why I had given up and decided to live with my illness.

Thank you so much for the results achieved.

With best wishes,

Walter Pierpaoli

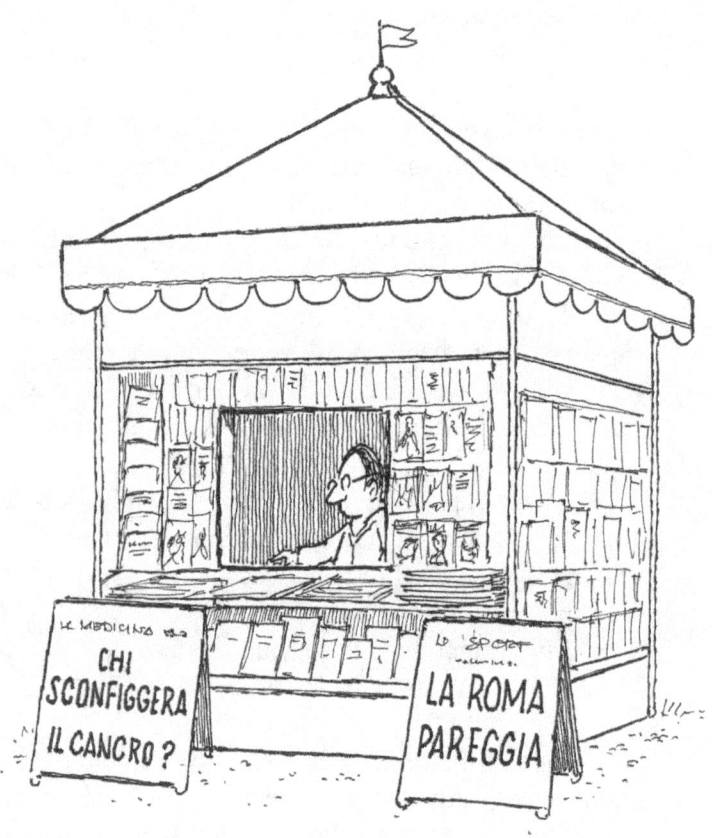

XXVI. Your treatment is phenomenal!

Dear Doctor Pierpaoli,

I wanted to let you know that there are now only 7 days of life left in my kit! I wanted to thank you so much: my partner *S.* was right – your treatment is phenomenal! I sent you an email informing you that everything was going well except for the fact that I found it really difficult to wake up in the mornings; however, this problem has now gone away and I wake up feeling rested and perfectly ready to go. I have measured my temperature as soon as I wake up in the last 4 days: 36.0; 35.8; 35.8; 36.0. I started off with a body weight of 64.5 and I am now 63.3 but I think the fat removal has been positive (see my stomach!). My kit is number 2 with a Thyroid IBSA 125 tablet.

Thank you in advance for your kindness and I am eagerly looking forward to the new treatment you will prescribe for me.

Yours sincerely,

M.B.

* * *

That's fine; I will check and see to it. Your temperature is still low, if you are measuring it scrupulously. I would not change anything for now. Thank

Walter Pierpaoli

you for your trust in me; this is what my therapies are based on.
Yours sincerely,

Walter Pierpaoli

Thank you. I remember that I came to see you and I told you I felt my body was very depressed and this had repercussions also on my morale. I can now tell you that, especially in the last week, I have again felt the joy and enthusiasm that I used to have before, and this means a lot.
I measured my temperature with an old mercury thermometer before getting out of bed, as soon as I woke up, for five minutes. I hope I did right...
With best wishes, and again many thanks,

M.B.

*

Dear Doctor Pierpaoli,

Your treatment is changing my quality of life; it is ages since I felt so strong, even right into the late evening. In the mornings I have a lot of difficulty waking up but I am sure that this is because my body-system just needs a little time, and that it is on the way to being cured... it is only just over a month since I started!...
Thank you again!
Yours sincerely,

M.B.

XXVII: In support of a new doctor-patient alliance

Dear Doctor,

I am touched by your thanks but, believe me, people with your charisma and your magnetism arouse interest and a sense of involvement not just in me, but in all those who are able to recognize the rare pearls in life. And there is so much willingness to help, kindness, sacrifice and love for science – uncommon qualities in an age of egoism and materialism, where the only things of value are those that can be taken to the bank!

As regards the analyses I have decided to send you straight away those we already have available, because they date back to just a few days ago.

However, if you think it appropriate to repeat them, or require any other particular type of examination, please let me know and I will arrange for them immediately.

With admiration,

O.D.

Walter Pierpaoli

PAEDIATRICIAN

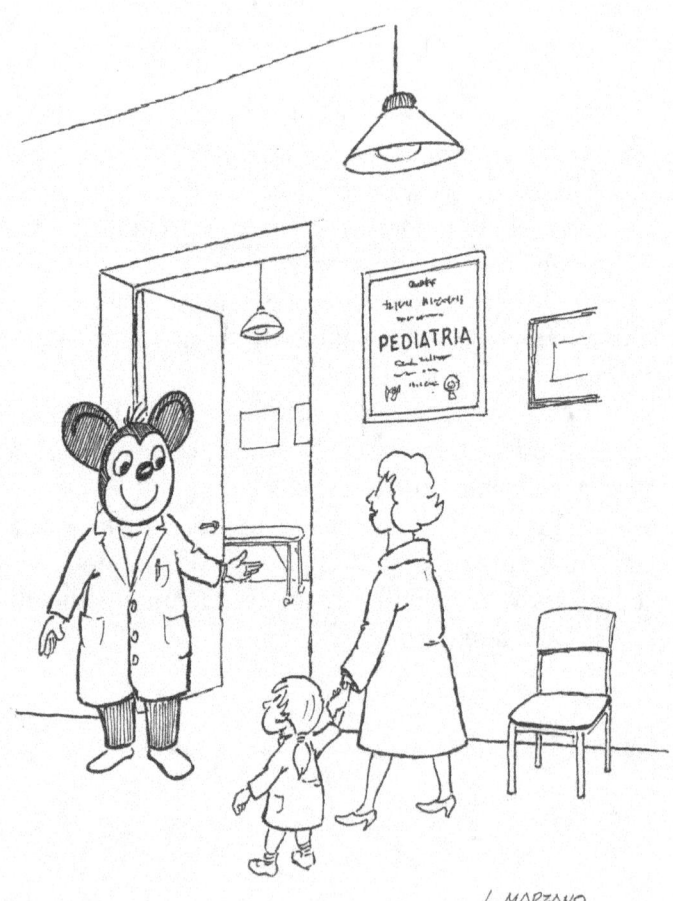

XXVIII. Caring for the body and caring for the soul

Dear Doctor,

Please allow me to send you my thanks. You follow the progress of your patients with such affection, treating their souls as well as their bodies and inspiring reflection on the values of life, which have perhaps been put to one side by some people and at times, forgotten. Youth is not a period of life, it is a state of mind that consists of a certain form of will, a disposition of the imagination and an emotive force; it is boldness prevailing over timidity and a thirst for adventure over comfort. We do not get older simply because we have lived for a certain number of years, but only when we abandon our ideals. Being young means still having, at the age of sixty or seventy, one's love for what is marvellous, amazement at what is sparkling and for bright thoughts, an intrepid attention to events, the insatiable desire of the child for everything that is new, and the sense of the delightful side of existence. We will stay young as long as our hearts are able to receive the messages of beauty, boldness, courage, greatness and strength that reach us from the earth, from a person or from infinity. When all the fibres of our heart are broken and the snows of pessimism and the ice of cynicism have accumulated on them, only then will we become old: may God have mercy on our souls.

I wish you, who are like a father to me, best wishes for the New Year.

With kind regards,

P.S

Walter Pierpaoli

XXIX. Treating multiple sclerosis

Dear Doctor,

I am writing to record my 'misadventure' with multiple sclerosis. It is an evil term, and difficult to accept; but this is not how you saw it, when I met you thanks to the open-mindedness and the courage of the doctor who was attending me. It all goes back to 2001, with the paresthesia of my whole right side, difficulties in walking and uncontrolled movement of my right arm and difficulties in speech. Tired of all the medical visits and tired of treatments that offered no prospect of recovery and with many, too many certainties in the contraindications, I decided to meet you. Twelve years have passed since then and I feel fine; if it had not been for your constant dedication, I would not find myself today calmly tackling life and work. I hope many other people make the same choice as me. I wish you again a long life, full of satisfaction.

R.

Dr. A….. M…..
PSYCHIATRY

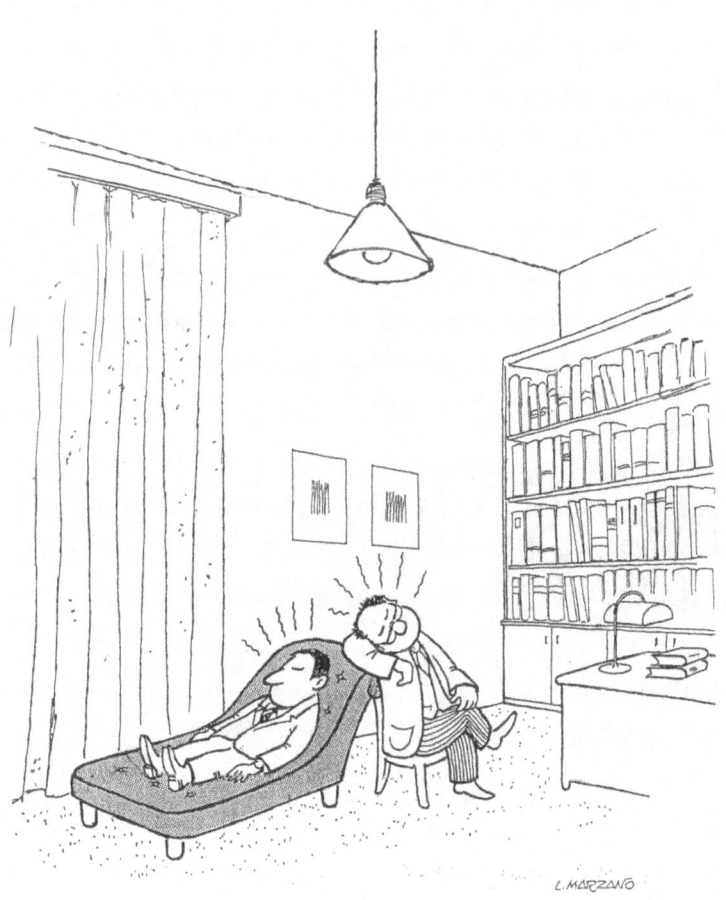

Walter Pierpaoli

XXX. Regularity regained

Dear Doctor Pierpaoli,

I am writing to give you good news, which is that my intestine has gone back to being regular. In addition, for the first time in years, my menstrual cycle has shown the first losses on the 27th day and, in the days of intense flow, I have not had any strong pains and therefore have not needed to take painkillers. Although the joint pains in my hands and feet are still there, I think this is a first step forward! As far as the chest pains are concerned, I think they are closely linked to my emotional state and I see it as an area of muscular contraction, to the extent that I often feel the need to expand my chest to relieve the tension.

I also wanted to inform you that after the intestinal problems I lost a few kilos in weight and so far I have not put them on again, but I have to say that I do not feel weak or lacking in energy.

Since 22 December – that is, when you prescribed it for me – I have been taking ¾ of Thyroid IBSA 125 and I attach my basal metabolic rate which I continue to measure even though not actually every day.

Finally, I would like to ask you for some information concerning my husband, since he has just started reading your book and I was wondering if he, too, could take melatonin – and if so, for how long and in what doses.

I look forward to hearing from you.
With best wishes,

S.S.

Dear *S.*,

Thank you for your fruitful collaboration. I always expect this kind of news from those who return carefully to an even balance. Go on and certainly give a tablet to your husband, too, so that you will not lose him prematurely. Women, as well as being more flexible and intelligent and long-lived, have also understood what I do and therefore they will further enlarge the distance between them and male creatures who, basically, after their necessary role in procreation, are useful for what? I am joking but there is a certain truth in this, don't you think?

With very best wishes,

Walter Pierpaoli

Walter Pierpaoli

XXXI. Farewell, pain!

Dear Doctor,

I wanted to start off by thanking you because I have felt like a new person since I have been taking your treatment: I have much less pain and I am able to do things that I could not before even have imagined I would go back to doing. I felt like a sixty-year-old woman who could not even make the minimum of effort because pains kept her in bed for the whole of the following day; now, however, I feel really much better and having days without pain is magnificent.

After we were in touch three weeks ago I measured my temperature and it was still 35.8. As you advised me, I increased the Thyroid IBSA 125 by half a tablet. I will finish the tablets in a week's time: my temperature fluctuates between 36.2 and 36.4. If I need to give you any other information, please let me know!

With very best wishes,

S.R.

ORGAN TRANSPLANTS

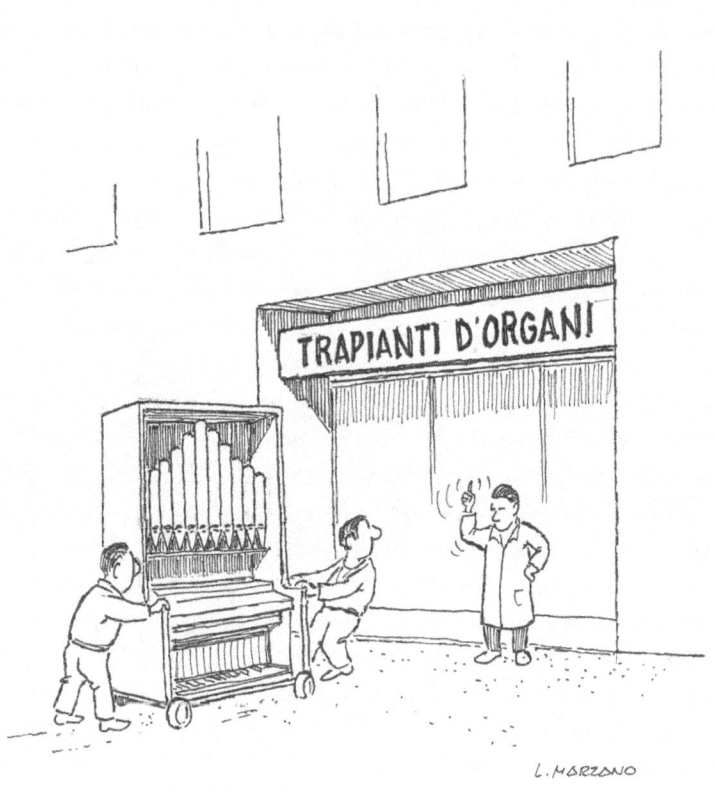

Walter Pierpaoli

XXXII. My health is just great!!!

Dear Doctor Pierpaoli,

I have finished the last kit you prescribed for me. Would you please be so kind as to send me a prescription for the new one? Yesterday I had a sudden thought: I have not had the slightest worsening of my condition since 2006. I was really lucky to meet you...
Best wishes,

T.P.

*

Dear Doctor,

I hope everything is going well. My health is just GREAT!!! I am taking this opportunity to let you know that I am getting married on the first of May.
I have also finished the kit you prescribed, so I am looking forward to my new prescription.
Yours sincerely,

T.P.

* * *

I will do that, and many congratulations and best wishes for your happiness in these difficult times… Send me a photo of your wedding afterwards. Thank you,

Walter Pierpaoli

I certainly will! You have made this happy occasion possible… I will never be able to thank you enough…

T.P.

Walter Pierpaoli

XXXIII. Just a matter of luck?

Dear Doctor Pierpaoli,

I am writing to tell you that, for the second year running, my condition is stable. Thank you very much! There was a slight worsening, but it was practically insignificant according to the oculist who also told me I can count myself lucky. To this I replied that it was not just a matter of luck; behind it there is a continuous work of immunology and Shiatsu and acupuncture; there is a healthy diet and there are your treatments – but unfortunately there was no dialogue to be had with him… Just a kind of amazement, if nothing else!

Regarding the Thyroid IBSA 125, in your prescription you prescribed one tablet per day for me. Well, around two months ago, when my temperature went down, you advised me to go up to one and a half. I am reporting my temperature for the last 10 days, so that you will know how to advise me: 36.4; 36.1; 35.9: 36; 36.1; 36.5; 36.5; 36.6; 36.2; 36.2. Thank you for everything and best wishes,

Z.

*

Dear Dr. Pierpaoli,

I am writing to let you know that the result of the sight test was EXCELLENT, in the sense that the test done now, compared with the one last year, showed no worsening, and there was even a slight improvement! I think this is important; the oculist was slightly puzzled, attributing the positive result to greater attention on my part during the test. But in general terms he confirmed that there has been a slight improvement. Moreover, I myself compared the two previous sight tests and I noted that the improvement was much more contained; in those cases, yes, it might have been attributable to a state of greater concentration on my part. And anyway, the important fact is that there has been no deterioration. THANK YOU! I am going on with your kits and I am also continuing, as I have done for two years now, with the specific monthly Shiatsu treatments, taking advantage of the help of a dear friend who does it for love – and (I am sure!) I can say the same for you.

Goodbye, and thank you again for everything.

Z.

Walter Pierpaoli

XXXIV. Thank you Walter Pierpaoli!

The first time they talked to me about him I simply thought he must be a good doctor. I was at the osteopath's trying to understand what contracture was shortening my son's right limb and I was telling her about all the other problems affecting this little blond boy, bright and beautiful, with his green eyes.

His teachers admitted to me that when they had to tell him off for some misdemeanour (and he committed a lot of these, as well as avoiding doing boring homework) they could not do it. They inevitably relented when he looked at them with his big wide-open eyes. The little girls all played at being his 'girlfriend' and even the other mothers never failed always to pay me compliments.

Just like in *Dorian Gray*, with such a beautiful appearance one would never have suspected so many problems. At about eighteen months, he started with recurring coughs and bronchitis. The paediatrician, of course, after cough syrups and aerosols which had no benefit, moved on to antibiotics and bronchodilators, finishing up with cortisone: none of this was effective. We spent so many nights walking around with the child's head on our shoulder, one hand on his back so that we could feel those wheezing bronchial tubes carrying at least a small amount of oxygen... When he was lying down, the cough suffocated him. Then he reverted to being the little monkey he had always been, jumping around, running and having fun with his pals.

I explained to my friend the osteopath that when the paediatrician had started to talk about asthmatic cough and rheumatic fever I had got frightened and my husband and I had decided to take him to a specialist in immunology.

The immunologist waited for the following attack, he prescribed tests and spirometry (which was to be continued at home as well) and then he gave us antibiotics and cortisone again, urging us to come back when the child had recovered through the 'therapy'.

The therapy in question consisted of giving a minimum dose of cortisone with a pre-dosed inhaler, morning and evening for at least one year because, by doing so, there was the possibility of preventing the attacks and the total amount of cortisone would surely be less than that of a shock therapy, and the side effects would also be reduced.

I certainly did not, at that time, realise the damage that cortisone might create, even though I had always been worried by this drug. The damage it would cause to my son's physical development was still more frightening: according to the immunologist, the boy would grow a little less than the height established by his DNA, and since I am one metre fifty-one and my husband is one sixty-eight, how 'tall' would our son become?

'OK', I told myself regretfully: health comes first. He has not had any more asthma attacks, but he always had a blocked nose, and he could have up to ten series of sneezes when he woke up. If he spent an afternoon playing in the countryside, he would certainly cough all night!

And what about the high temperatures? Every two or three weeks I was unable to make him get up in the mornings; he felt ill, he had a headache, maybe he had

been coughing and sneezing the whole night long. He missed school and then, in the afternoon, he went back to being full of energy. Of course, I thought he was kidding me; but if I insisted I realised that, once he was up, he was really weak; anyway, his high temperature was real, his lymph-nodes always enlarged and his face pale.

When he was about ten, I noticed that the small scratches he got while playing, instead of clearing up, tended to produce pus and to increase in size. A scab on his knees became a nightmare, it would not heal! The small bottles of Mercurochrome were quickly used up but the wounds were slow to heal. So we went onto antibiotic ointments and medicated plasters.

We repeated the tests for the umpteenth time: the antistreptolysin O test was always between positive and negative, but all the other values seemed to be normal and they did not know what to do.

The osteopath said to me: 'Well why don't you try contacting Pierpaoli? A friend of mine was happy with his treatment; I'll get the telephone number for you tomorrow! I told myself that there was no harm in trying.

When I heard him talk I understood that he was an excellent doctor. I took the number and got ready with the words I would have to say to get an urgent appointment. It was not the secretary who answered, as I had expected, but Dr. Pierpaoli himself; I could not get the words out and, stammering, I tried to explain to him the reason for my call.

'Have my secretary give you the fax number for the analyses and take his basal temperature. When we meet

I'll have a clear picture, since you'll have given me a preview of the results by fax.'

This was very decisive!

As soon as I got the results of the tests and when I had taken the first temperatures, I sent the fax and Pierpaoli replied within a few days!

I still lovingly keep the fax: 'I'll tell you what I would do if he were my son or my nephew... I don't know what therapies he has undergone, (however, I can imagine quite clearly...): perhaps a lot of antibiotics and cortisone. I'm afraid there might be an immune-depressive state based on a thyroid alteration. It's a question here of gently and skilfully aiding growth and development without causing damage'. I started to warm to him. Then he started talking about kits, Thyroid IBSA 125, Lugol, DHEA, Algae and a lot of vitamins, as well as the essential Melatonin ZN-SE. 'I think the boy will react well. Give him a varied diet but keep to normal mealtimes and we'll be in touch again in about a month.'

I was bewildered by the assortment of new terms I had to deal with, but I got moving and after a few days, the package arrived and everything was ready on a tray with explanatory notes for the daily therapy: years of assisting my mother who was cardiopathic, hypertensive and at the limit of dialysis because of chronic renal failure came in useful, unfortunately, for something...

Walter Pierpaoli

Ten days later, in the car, my son suddenly exclaimed: 'Mum, do you know I feel really well?'

I was a bit surprised. What did that mean? I did not imagine there was anything that would bring such an

immediate benefit that it could be detected by a little twelve-year-old boy! He confirmed it again: he felt well!

When I met him I was charmed. We arrived at the appointment feeling definitely cheered up. The doctor explained to us what might have happened to our son's immune system and then showed us his way of working. It was not the classic examination on the couch, but rather a nice, long chat with a lot of wise advice.

Four years have passed since then. Our boy is now sixteen, and is one metre eighty tall. He has a good dose of 'flu almost every year, but he has not had any more low-grade fevers. He has only missed the days at school that he wanted to miss and he still has some remaining allergy. But all the other problems, (apart from the usual ones of adolescence which are always a problem for parents!) have disappeared. In the meantime, both my two daughters and I myself are following the doctor's treatment. I have bothered him so many times! Now we know that, genetically, we are predisposed to hypothyroidism. But that is another story.

With many thanks to Doctor Pierpaoli!
(signed letter)

By way of conclusion

The patient and I, I and the patient

Walter Pierpaoli

If I forget everything I have heard about the doctor-patient relationship and refer to my decades of experience as a freelance doctor, outside the 'health system' -both in Italy and in Switzerland – and therefore as a researcher who, in over 40 years of intense research in all medical disciplines, (from immunology to endocrinology and from psycho-neuro-immunology to oncology and so on), who has developed his own therapies, avoiding recourse to drugs except in rare cases of bacterial infections – I can only be appalled at what I have seen and heard and still see today. Nowadays, there is a 'shredder system' in place, which ignores the feelings and the sensitivity of the human being and the close link that must exist between doctors and patients – or *those assumed to be so.*

The brutalisation of medicine is the outcome of socio-economic changes and the pervasive, ever-present domination of money as the preponderant element in medicine. This is not a subject that concerns me, as I believe the situation to be beyond all control: in one sense it should be simply *ignored.* Moreover, even doctors are now enslaved by their 'employers', who may be easily identified.

I therefore think I should explain briefly my attitude and how I *feel* the relationship with those who apply to me and ask for help. I must stress that this relationship, developed over time, from my awareness as a doctor who, while using notions he has collected over the decades, has created a completely new and personal 'therapeutic world', based on his personal discoveries and observations, without allowing himself to be contaminated by fashions and exaggerated and misleading statements from the pharmaceutical industry, which reflect the spirit of profit *at any cost.*

1. If I am not able to identify with the patient who is really suffering, or who only believes he or she is suffering; if I am not in a position to give my close attention to what he or she is saying; if I am 'in a hurry' and 'snowed under with work'; well, if I am all these things, I am not in a position to practise medicine. People who ask me for help and, at the end of their tether, put their lives in my hands, must be able to count on me, always and until they are cured or reach a state of balance.

2. The patient must be given elementary teaching, which is part of a heritage of ancient wisdom that has been lost since the end of the Second World War. This is why I drafted a set of reflections published in *The ageless man* (Morlacchi Editore, Perugia 2010). Pathologies very often arise not so much from the genetic make-up that each of us carries around from birth, but rather from an incorrect and damaging lifestyle. It seems incredible how an adverse environment has been created without us realising it! The changes taking place around the population, which is undergoing assault from harmful molecules and gases and is not aware of what is happening to it (and is not even interested in knowing!), are nothing less than horrific. But we do not see the danger except when we are ill. And illness rarely leads us to reform our lifestyle; on the contrary, resignation sets in, leading to the false belief that everything has gone wrong and is inescapable.

3. Those who come to see me for the first time and arrive after numerous therapeutic failures are led to rethink and feel 'shocked' at everything that has happened to them. The glimmer of hope for a possible cure, in fact, produces a radical change. This effect must certainly not be linked to illusions and false hopes, but to the charge of optimism and faith that generates in the patient a genuine psychosomatic reconversion, which is visible already after just a few minutes. Hope, together with the vital charge that the doctor must instil, go to create what I would call, in psycho-neuro-endocrinological terms *radical restructuring of the awareness of self and of one's own body.*

4. In spite of this doctor-patient relationship being extremely complex and also exhausting for those who are trying to manage the health of others, I must stress that many components coexist within it, that each clinical case is unique and there is no repetitiveness: each life reflects a multitude of genetic and environmental components. The bond between genetics and environment, (nutrition, family, work, habits) makes up a unique example and therefore each patient is a completely *new* case. There are however, common components of a physiological nature, since there is repetitiveness in the biological structure of the body, which obeys the laws of the Cosmos and of the Planetary System- in which life itself was generated.

5. I also wanted to say that one must not confuse the concept of charity and mercy, however praiseworthy, with

that pervasive and innate sense of *pietas*, which is engaging in each human being and which knows no

boundaries either of territory or ethnic group. This sense of sharing sufferings, deeply rooted in the Greco-Roman culture and deeply expressed in the sense of spontaneous solidarity, (in which I identify myself, for example, with the deep humanity of Russian literature), comprises the basis for the doctor-patient relationship, in my opinion.

6. The 'doctor's triumph' is to see his or her patient cured. We delude ourselves if we think that there are more gratifying rewards! That love we always talk about, without knowing how it should be defined, shows itself then. If ever love generates love, as the great Erich Fromm emphasised, the doctor's dedication to the psychic and somatic health of the patient gives the real sense of humanity, once doctor and patient meet to share the joy of feeling healthy and well.

Walter Pierpaoli

Walter Pierpaoli

HOSPITAL

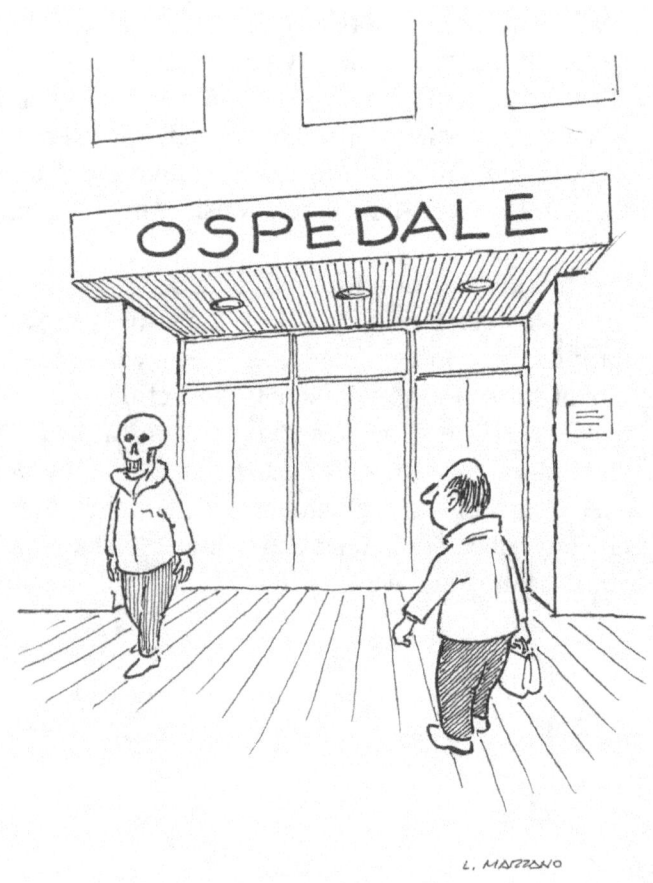

Afterword

I have known Walter Pierpaoli as a scientist and as a man for several years. Right from the start I was fascinated by his profile as an independent researcher 'standing out from the crowd', always able to offer a practical, minimalist and synthetic interpretation of scientific knowledge. His is a vision far away from the self-celebratory view, full of advertising, that is so frequent in many areas of research where they often proclaim revolutionary discoveries that, after a few years, fall into the oblivion of useless things or are part of an infinite analytical jigsaw puzzle of little pieces of information, comprising an unknown whole.

Biology, physiology and physiopathology are at the centre of Pierpaoli's wisdom, contrary in principle to pharmaceutical chemistry and to medicine understood as the simple treating of the symptom, which is the final expression of the pathological process. Research has led him, as a scientist, during long and exciting years of experimentation, to interpret the biological keys of the chronic diseases linked to ageing and vice versa. These are, in fact the result of the neuro-immuno-endocrine system progressively losing its control and guidance of the organism. This 'de-regulation' is in part genetically determined but often accelerated and modified by acquired variables such as pollution, lifestyle, diet, etc. Pierpaoli's research has thus allowed him to understand and interpret what effect the deterioration of regular biological processes has on the health of our body. The genetic program established at birth – growth, development, reproduction, ageing and death – can, in fact, be partly modified in a quantitative and qualitative sense. This can be seen as a 're-regulation' of the neuro-pineal axis, of the pituitary hypothalamus system and so mediated by the peripheral immunoendocrine system. The end result is intended to be the restoration of the natural and non-pathological ageing process, free from chronic-degenerative diseases.

His experimental research has taken Pierpaoli around the world. For forty years, he has worked for laboratories of great prestige. Finally he has added a piece of the mosaic that is generally missing in the life of a modern scientist: translating the knowledge acquired into clinical practice. This aspect brings Pierpaoli closer to the figure of the Renaissance man of science where, in the same person, the boundaries between observation, innovation and practical application were removed.

The functioning of the pineal gland, the role of melatonin, resetting the neuroendocrine axis, defining the molecules essential for the balance of life and cell survival have as their ultimate aim the defeat of ageing understood as illness, decline, deterioration and invalidity, the contrasting of degenerative diseases and the improvement of quality of life.

As well as being a great scientist, Walter is also and above all a doctor and he has never forgotten this. His curiosity, the desire to put into practice in the first person what he has learnt from his research over the years, have been the catalyst that has driven him on to carry out his clinical work.

His view of the patient is different: it springs from the awareness of the reversibility of chronic degenerative diseases connected to ageing and therefore to the reversal of ageing itself, which is made to come within the natural program of genetic expectation.

His clinical view, therefore, is light years in advance of the pharmacocentric view of current medicine, which catalogues and controls *pharmacologically*, without ever curing them, chronic diseases such as diabetes, atherosclerosis, arterial hypertension and in general all diseases caused by a metabolic disorder. The result of all this is that people often survive and grow old in chronic depression, taking more than ten different drugs a day, for all the rest of their lives. The penalty for interrupting the drug is the uncontrolled resumption of the disease.

The patient who, during the past years, has taken advantage of Pierpaoli's *biological-re-educational* medicine (*biological-re-educational* in the sense of re-establishing normal metabolic functions and therefore the correct functioning of the systemic biology), rediscovers the feeling of well-being that only a real restoring to health can give. The letters from these patients are the most symbolic representation of this. The educational books *The key of life* and *The ageless man* are the earlier works in the trilogy that concludes with *Happy Patients*: now, finally, we see at first hand the clinical results of the discoveries made by this man of science.

Valerio di Nicola
MD, PhD, Consultant of General and Colorectal Surgery,
Noble's Hospital, IOM (UK)

Walter Pierpaoli

Contents